DIABETES MASTERING COOKBOOK

introduction to diabetes with easy and healthy
diabetics recipes

Dr.James L.Gonzalez.

Table of contents

Chapter 1

What is Diabetes?:

Diabetes is a typical condition that influences individuals, everything being equal. There are a few types of diabetes. Type 2 is the most well-known. A blend of treatment methodologies can assist you with dealing with the condition to carry on with a solid life and forestall confusion.

Diabetes is a condition that happens when your glucose (glucose) is excessively high. It creates when your pancreas doesn't make sufficient insulin or any whatsoever, or when your body isn't answering the impacts of insulin appropriately.

Diabetes influences individuals, all things considered. Most types of diabetes are ongoing

(long-lasting), and all structures are reasonable with drugs as well as way of life change
Glucose (sugar) predominantly comes from starches in your food and beverages. It's your body's go-to wellspring of energy. Your blood conveys glucose to all your body's cells to use for energy.

At the point when glucose is in your circulation system, it needs assistance — a "key" — to arrive at its last objective. This key is insulin (a chemical). On the off chance that your pancreas isn't making sufficient insulin or your body isn't utilizing it appropriately, glucose develops in your circulatory system, causing high glucose (hyperglycemia).

After some time, having reliably high blood glucose can cause medical conditions, for example, coronary illness, nerve harm, and eye issues.

The specialized name for diabetes will be diabetes mellitus. Another condition shares the expression "diabetes" — diabetes insipidus — yet they're unmistakable. They share the name "diabetes" since the two of them cause expanded thirst and successive pee. Diabetes insipidus is a lot more uncommon than diabetes mellitus.

What are the kinds of diabetes:
There are a few kinds of diabetes. The most widely recognized structures include:

Type 2 diabetes: With this sort of, your body doesn't make sufficient insulin as well as your body's cells don't respond regularly to the insulin (insulin obstruction). This is the most widely recognized sort of diabetes. It fundamentally influences grown-ups, yet kids can have it also.
Prediabetes: This type is the stage before Type 2 diabetes. Your blood glucose levels are higher than ordinary yet not sufficiently high to be authoritatively determined to have Type 2 diabetes.
Type 1 diabetes: This type is an immune system illness wherein your safe framework assaults and obliterates insulin-delivering cells in your

pancreas for obscure reasons. Up to 10% of individuals who have diabetes have Type 1. It's typically analyzed in kids and youthful grown-ups, however, it can be created at whatever stage in life.

Gestational diabetes: This type is created in certain individuals during pregnancy. Gestational diabetes generally disappears after pregnancy. In any case, in the event that you have gestational diabetes, you're at a higher gamble of creating Type 2 diabetes further down the road.

Different kinds of diabetes include:

Type 3c diabetes: This type of diabetes happens when your pancreas encounters harm (other than immune system harm), which influences its capacity to deliver insulin. Pancreatitis, pancreatic disease, cystic fibrosis, and hemochromatosis can all prompt pancreas harm that causes diabetes. Having your pancreas eliminated (pancreatectomy) additionally brings about Type 3c.

Idle immune system diabetes in grown-ups (LADA): Like Sort 1 diabetes, LADA additionally results from an immune system response, however, it grows significantly more leisurely than Type 1. Individuals determined to have LADA are generally beyond 30 years old.

Development beginning diabetes of the youthful (MODY): MODY, likewise called monogenic diabetes, occurs because of an acquired hereditary transformation that influences how your body makes and uses insulin. There are as of now north of 10 unique kinds of MODY. It influences up to 5% of individuals with diabetes and ordinarily runs in families.

Neonatal diabetes: This is an intriguing type of diabetes that happens within the initial half year of life. It's likewise a type of monogenic diabetes. Around half of the children with neonatal diabetes have the deep-rooted structure called super durable neonatal diabetes mellitus. For the other portion, the condition vanishes within a couple of months from the beginning, however, it can return sometime down the road. This is called transient neonatal diabetes mellitus.

Fragile diabetes: Weak diabetes is a type of Type 1 diabetes that is set apart by continuous and extreme episodes of high and low glucose level This insecurity frequently prompts hospitalization. In uncommon cases, a pancreas relocation might be important to treat weak diabetes forever.

Symptoms & Causes of Diabetes;
Side effects of diabetes include:
Expanded thirst (polydipsia) and dry mouth.
Successive pee.
Weakness.
Obscured vision.
Unexplained weight reduction.
Deadness or shivering in your grasp or feet.
Slow-recuperating bruises or cuts.
Successive skin or potentially vaginal yeast contaminations.
It's vital to converse with your medical services supplier assuming you or your kid has these side effects.

Extra insights regarding side effects per kind of diabetes include:

Type 1 diabetes: Side effects of T1D can grow rapidly — more than half a month or months.

You might foster extra side effects that are indications of a serious inconvenience called diabetes-related ketoacidosis (DKA). DKA is hazardous and requires prompt clinical treatment. DKA side effects incorporate retching, stomach torments, fruity-smelling breath, and working relaxation.

Type 2 diabetes and prediabetes: You might not have any side effects whatsoever, or you may not see them since they grow gradually. Routine blood work may show a high glucose level before you perceive side effects. One more conceivable indication of prediabetes is obscured skin on specific pieces of your body (acanthosis nigricans).

Gestational diabetes: You regularly won't see side effects of gestational diabetes. Your medical care supplier will test you for gestational diabetes somewhere in the range of 24 and 28 weeks of pregnancy.

What causes diabetes?
An excessive amount of glucose circling in your circulation system causes diabetes, no matter what the sort. Notwithstanding, the motivation behind why your blood glucose levels are high varies depending upon the sort of diabetes.

Causes of diabetes include:

Insulin obstruction: Type 2 diabetes primarily results from insulin opposition. Insulin obstruction happens when cells in your muscles, fat, and liver don't answer as they ought to insulin. A few factors and conditions add to shifting levels of insulin obstruction, including weight, absence of active work, diet, hormonal uneven characteristics, hereditary qualities, and certain meds.

Immune system sickness: Type 1 diabetes and LADA happen when your resistant framework goes after the insulin-delivering cells in your pancreas.

Hormonal awkward nature: During pregnancy, the placenta discharges chemicals that cause insulin obstruction. You might foster gestational diabetes if your pancreas can't deliver sufficient insulin obstruction. Other chemical-related conditions like acromegaly and Cushing disorder can likewise cause Type 2 diabetes.

Pancreatic harm: Actual harm to your pancreas — from a condition, medical procedure, or injury — can affect its capacity to make insulin, bringing about Type 3c diabetes.

Hereditary changes: Certain hereditary transformations can cause MODY and neonatal diabetes.

Long haul utilization of specific meds can likewise prompt Sort 2 diabetes, including HIV/Helps meds and corticosteroids.

Risk Factors for Type 2 Diabetes

Risk Elements for Type 2 Diabetes
Type 2 diabetes is accepted to have areas of strength for a connection, implying that it will in general disagree families. If you have a parent, sibling, or sister who has it, your possibilities rise. A few qualities might be connected with type 2 diabetes. Get some information about a diabetes test if you have any of the accompanying gambling factors:

Hypertension
High blood fatty substance (fat) levels. It's excessively high if it's north of 150 milligrams for every deciliter (mg/dL).
Low "great" cholesterol level. It's excessively low assuming it's under 40 mg/dL.
Gestational diabetes or bringing forth a child weighing more than 9 pounds

Prediabetes. That implies your glucose level is better than average, however, you don't have the sickness yet.

Coronary illness

High-fat and carb diet. This can some of the time be the consequence of food weakness when you don't approach sufficient good food.

High liquor consumption

A stationary way of life

Heftiness or being overweight

Polycystic ovary disorder (PCOS)

Being of an identity that is at higher gamble: African Americans, Local Americans, Hispanic Americans, and Asian Americans are bound to get type 2 diabetes than non-Hispanic whites.

You're more than 45 years old. More seasoned age is a critical gambling factor for type 2 diabetes. The gamble of type 2 diabetes starts to rise altogether around age 45 and rises significantly after age 65.

You've had an organ relocated. After an organ relocates, you want to consume medications until the end of your life so your body doesn't dismiss the contributor organ. These medications help organ transfers succeed, however, a large number of them, for example, tacrolimus (Astagraf, Prograf) or steroids, can cause diabetes or make it worse. A legitimate eating routine and sound way of life propensities, alongside prescription, on the off chance that you want it, can assist you with overseeing type 2 diabetes the same way you oversee different parts of your life. Make certain to look for the most recent data on this condition as you become your well-being advocate.

The Job of Insulin in the Reason for Type 2 Diabetes

To comprehend the reason why insulin is significant, it assists with finding out how your body involves nourishment for energy. Your body is composed of millions of cells. To make energy, these cells need food in an exceptionally straightforward structure. At the point when you eat or drink, a significant part of the food is separated into a straightforward sugar called glucose. It travels through your circulation system to these cells, where it gives the energy your body needs for day-to-day exercises.

Insulin and different chemicals control how much glucose is in your circulation system. Your pancreas is continuously delivering modest quantities of insulin. At the point when how much glucose in your blood ascends to a specific level, the pancreas will deliver more insulin to drive more glucose into the cells. This causes the glucose levels in the blood (blood glucose levels) to drop.

To keep blood glucose levels from getting excessively low (hypoglycemia, or low glucose), your body signals you to eat and lets some glucose out of the stores kept in the liver. It likewise advises the body to deliver less insulin. People with diabetes either don't create insulin or their body's cells can never again utilize their insulin. This prompts high blood sugar. By definition, diabetes is:

A blood glucose level of more prominent than or equivalent to 126 milligrams for every deciliter (mg/dL) of blood following an 8-hour quick (not eating anything)

A non-fasting glucose level more prominent than or equivalent to 200 mg/dL, alongside side effects of diabetes

A glucose level more noteworthy than or equivalent to 200 mg/dL on a 2-hour glucose resilience test

A1c is more prominent than or equivalent to 6.5%. Except if the individual is having clear side effects of diabetes or is in a diabetic emergency, the finding should be affirmed with a recurrent test.

Insulin, Medicines, & Other Diabetes Treatments;

Diabetes is a difficult condition that is welcomed by diminished insulin emission from the pancreas and lessened insulin responsiveness in the muscle cells. It is portrayed by unreasonable pee, outrageous thirst, high glucose, and expanded appetite.1

There are various meds available to assist with dealing with this condition, however, coming up next is the main 10 as far as showing viability in bringing down A1C and glucose levels
1. Insulin (long-and quick acting)

Patients with type 1 diabetes (T1D) should be treated with insulin, as the beta cells in their pancreas never again produce it. Insulin assumes an essential part in glucose take-up and is expected by the muscle and fat tissue.2 In any case, insulin isn't exclusively for patients with T1D; those with type 2 diabetes (T2D) may likewise be put on insulin, however, by and large solely after neglecting to reach glycemic focuses after being put on various oral specialists for quite a while. Patients with diabetes commonly get different infusions each day, including bolus insulin managed before dinners and the long-acting basal insulin that brings down glucose levels over the long haul. Insulin is delegated a high-risk drug since it can make patients experience hypoglycemia, however, the advantages of this treatment offset the dangers.

The most well-known insulins I see endorsed in my everyday practice are Basaglar (long-acting) and NovoLog (fast acting

2. Metformin (biguanide class)

Metformin is viewed as the first-line oral specialist for patients with diabetes and can be utilized to treat pre-diabetes. It works by diminishing glucose creation in the liver, expanding insulin awareness, and bringing down gastrointestinal sugar retention. Metformin has been displayed to diminish A1 levels by 1% to 2%, fasting glucose levels by a normal of 25%, and postprandial glucose levels by 44%.3 Relying upon the seriousness of the condition, prescribers might attempt metformin joined with way-of-life alterations as monotherapy before adding more oral specialists to their patients' prescription regimens. The actual medication is very much endured, however before all else patients might encounter gastrointestinal steamed, like stomach squeezing, looseness of the bowels, and tooting.

3. Glipizide (sulfonylurea class)

If the A1C level isn't at focus following 3 months of utilizing metformin, a prescriber may then decide to add glipizide to a patient's routine.

This medicine works by animating insulin emission from the beta cells in the pancreas, which then, at that point, causes a reduction in postprandial blood glucose. Glipizide is utilized for the treatment of T2D; it is contraindicated in T1D because it can't be joined with insulin, which, as recently noted, is a necessary treatment for all T1D.

When joined with insulin, glipizide causes extreme hypoglycemia, which ought to be kept away from. The medication has been displayed to lessen A1C levels by 1% to 2% and works best when required 30 minutes before a meal.4 When on glipizide, a patient might encounter sickness and weight gain. The specialist is exceptionally viable, particularly at expanding insulin emission, however, its viability diminishes after long-haul use, as the beta cell capability might begin to decline.

4. Glimepiride (sulfonylurea class
Glimepiride works similarly to glipizide, yet isn't commonly joined with metformin as there is an expanded gamble of hypoglycemia when they are utilized together. Glimepiride is a once-everyday prescription and ought to be taken with the principal primary feast of the day. The medication works best when joined with a legitimate eating routine and exercise. Of the relative multitude of sulfonylureas, glimepiride is related to a minimal measure of weight gain and is liked for patients with cardiovascular sickness, as it comes up short on harming impacts on ischemic preconditioning.

5. Invokana (sodium-glucose cotransporter 2 inhibitor class)
On the off chance that a patient has a sulfa sensitivity the past 2 choices are not suit-capable, yet this one might be. Invokana works by hindering the sodium-glucose cotransporter 2 (SGLT2), which causes a decrease in the reabsorption of sifted glucose.

The medication additionally makes the patient discharge an abundance of glucose through their pee, bringing down plasma glucose fixations generally. This prescription has been displayed to bring down A1C levels by 0.7% to 1% yet is especially preferred by most patients in light of the critical weight reduction it can achieve.

There are a couple of disadvantages to Invokana, be that as it may, as it expands thirst and pee. Patients may likewise encounter more regular diseases, like urinary plot contaminations (UTIs), due to how much sugar is being discharged in their pee; as we probably are aware, microscopic organisms love sugar.

This prescription is additionally habitually matched with metformin and has its blend drug available called Invokamet, which can be expensive. Patients can find coupons for Invokana on the producer's site, which might make treatment more reasonable on the off chance that they qualify.

6. Jardiance (SGLT2 class)

Jardiance works similarly to Invokana, however, might be the favored choice in patients with a renal disability as it lessens the gamble for new or demolishing kidney sickness by 39%.3 In clinical preliminaries, Jardiance additionally exhibited diminished hospitalization rates from the cardiovascular breakdown in no less than 40% of patients, which is something to remember while choosing which SGLT2 is best for every patient.

7. Januvia (dipeptidyl peptidase 4 inhibitors)

Januvia works by managing blood glucose levels by expanding the arrival of insulin from the beta cells and diminishing the discharge of glucagon. Januvia, at last, improves the body's growth. This medication has been displayed to diminish A1C levels by 0.5% to 0.8% and essentially decline postprandial blood glucose levels.4 It likewise is weight-impartial, which is an or more. Patients on Januvia might encounter edema, rash, and UTIs. Albeit the prescription can be exorbitant, coupons are generally accessible.

8. Pioglitazone (thiazolidinediones)

Pioglitazone works by expanding fringe insulin responsiveness. It likewise has been shown to diminish A1C levels by 0.5% to 1.4%.3 even though pioglitazone has generally excellent viability as far as getting patients to target, it isn't the most ideal choice for some since it can cause or worsen cardiovascular breakdown. Patients might encounter queasiness and stomach upset while taking this prescription.

9. Victoza (glucagon-like peptide 1 agonist)

Victoza works by diminishing glucagon discharge, expanding glucose insulin emission, and easing back gastric exhaustion. It is an everyday infusion given regardless of feasts. This choice has shown critical weight reduction in patients. Victoza has been displayed to diminish A1C levels by 0.5% to 1.1% and decrease post-prandial blood glucose.3 Patients might encounter queasiness, which is the essential unfavorable impact that has been accounted for, however, this is a very much endured infusion.

10. Trulicity (glucagon-like peptide 1 agonist)

This choice is somewhat new and before long might be liked over Victoza as it just should be infused one time per week. It tends to be exorbitant, notwithstanding. The medication works similarly to Victoza yet requires fewer infusions. Patients additionally will see weight reduction with this medicine, even though it can cause torment and aggravation in the pancreas.

Chapter 2

At the point when you're previously determined to have diabetes, your primary care physician will probably prescribe diet and way of life changes to assist you with dealing with your glucose. While medications, for example, insulin solutions might be required, diet and exercise alone can bring about critical advancement.

Many individuals stress that these progressions will be excessively intense and difficult to stay with. When done accurately, the eating regimen and exercise expected to oversee glucose needn't bother with being a burden. However, likewise, with all ways of life changes, some discipline will be required. Overseeing diabetes with diet and exercise
At the point when a sound body has a glucose level that is too high, the pancreas delivers a

chemical called insulin. This chemical is the very thing that lets your body know that it needs to utilize or store an overabundance of glucose.

Contingent upon the sort of diabetes, a diabetic's body either doesn't create sufficient insulin or doesn't answer the insulin all around ok. With the insulin not functioning as really as it ought to, changes in the eating regimen become important to assist with controlling those levels.

The practice assists individuals with diabetes in more ways than one and, explicitly, assists with controlling glucose by two systems. To start with, practice itself increases glucose take-up. Second, practice works on the body's aversion to insulin, permitting the chemical to go about its business more.

Practice additionally assists with overseeing risk factors. Being overweight is a gamble factor for type 2 diabetes, which can be improved by practicing and getting fitter. Diabetes is a gamble factor for some heart-related issues, and exercise assists with diminishing those dangers.

Sustenance for diabetes
While just diminishing glucose is one objective of a solid diabetic eating regimen, it isn't the one to focus on. How you eat likewise assumes a major part in how in danger you are for difficulties of diabetes, like coronary illness.

A balanced eating routine that spotlights legitimate nourishment in all cases will assist with decreasing glucose and the gamble of complexities from diabetes too. Eating appropriately implies eating the right food sources in satisfactory sums while staying away from undesirable food varieties.

We should investigate what that implies practically speaking.

Food sources to eat

Your body needs numerous nutrients, minerals, electrolytes, and different supplements to manage its different frameworks. Certain supplements are helpful to your cardiovascular framework, some for the safe framework, etc.

While everybody ought to endeavor to eat a reasonable feast that incorporates the suggested measure of this multitude of fundamental supplements, diabetes builds the gamble factors for the majority of different circumstances, making legitimate sustenance significantly more significant for the people who have it. A balanced eating regimen will incorporate food sources from every one of the nutrition classes:

Boring vegetables

Non Starchy vegetables

Natural products

Grains

Protein

Dairy
Food sources to keep away from
While there are a lot of supplements you ought to keep up with in your eating routine, there are a few food sources that ought to be kept away from. Not all that in food is smart for you, and a portion of the fixings in our food are effectively terrible. That doesn't imply that you can never have a treat, yet it implies that you should be aware of the number of these food varieties you're eating.

It's additionally critical to comprehend which of these food sources are important for limited quantities yet unsafe when eaten in enormous sums and the number of are best stayed away from out and out.

Undesirable fat
There are a lot of food varieties with heart-solid fats like Omega 3 and Omega 6. However, there are likewise food varieties with undesirable fats,

like soaked fat and trans fat. Restricting your admission of the last option can hold your cholesterol under wraps and your course sound.

Pungent food varieties

Sodium, viewed as salt, is a vital electrolyte. Be that as it may, a great many people get undeniably a greater amount of it than required. At the point when you get an excessive amount of salt, your pulse can raise, prompting other heart-wellbeing aftereffects.

Food varieties with added sugar

As a diabetic, we've proactively perceived how monitoring sugar admission is significant. Added sugars, like those in many desserts and sweet beverages, give practically no dietary benefit and can have hindering well-being impacts.

Liquor

While it's OK to have a little liquor, drinking an excess can influence your glucose levels. Specialists suggest something like one beverage each day for ladies and two beverages each day for men.

Timing your dinners:
The planning of your dinners might be essential to dealing with your diabetes. Whether this is valid relies upon the treatment plan you're on.

For instance, somebody on insulin or other diabetes medicine might encounter a drop in glucose after taking it. While this is the motivation behind the medication, you don't need your glucose to drop excessively low. Your primary care physician might advise you to design your dinners as per your medication timing to appropriately direct glucose.

Your treatment plan might try to be more unambiguous. Your medical services group might suggest you eat a specific measure of sugar at a specific time. To make the greater part of your eating regimen changes, make certain to examine the points of interest of how you ought to transform it with your primary care physician.

Practice for diabetes:
There are various objectives for working out. Certain individuals need to acquire muscle, get fitter, work on cardiovascular capability, etc. For diabetes, you don't have to zero in on any of those particular objectives.

Even though we've perceived how shedding pounds can assist with eliminating one of your gambling factors for type 2 diabetes, the essential concern is simply getting dynamic. The Public Foundation of Wellbeing suggests 30 minutes of activity at a moderate or more noteworthy force five days per week. Moderate force implies that it's difficult yet manageable.

Foster a daily practice:
Practically any kind of exercise you pick can get you into the moderate-force zone or above. Find a movement that you truly appreciate doing, conclude which days you need to exercise, and

attempt to construct an activity program around that.

By working out at around similar time consistently and arranging what your exercises will be quite a bit early, it'll be simpler for you to foster the propensity for practicing and transform it into an extremely durable yet charming new way of life.

Move gradually up:
Whichever kind of activity you choose to do, recollect that you don't need to begin at full power. While you ought to sort out as long as 30 minutes out of every day, five days per week, that may be an excessive amount of action for you in the first place. You can attempt 20 minutes every day, three times each week, or even less, and add to it as you adapt.

Recollect that a little activity is superior to no activity. Do what feels great while provoking yourself to do somewhat more for a large number of days or many weeks until you hit the objective movement level.

Mix it up:
Doing a likewise exercise routine consistently until the end of your life is sufficient to make anybody tired of activity and surrender. That is the reason it's smart to trade out your schedules like clockwork and take a stab at a genuinely new thing. This can mean another weightlifting standard, an alternate sort of cardio, or anything you desire it to be.

Making a dinner plan:
Any new change in way of life is more straightforward if you make an arrangement and foster a propensity. Carving out an opportunity to foster a feast plan will provide you with a superior thought of the sorts of changes you want to make, yet will likewise make it simpler to adhere to the progressions step by step than attempting to sort it out on the fly.

By preparing, you can carve out the opportunity to guarantee every feast will have the supplements your body needs and assist with keeping you inside your glucose targets. There are two significant techniques prescribed to individuals with diabetes for controlling their glucose levels: counting sugars and the plate strategy.

Understanding part size:
Before we discuss both strategies, we should initially carve out an opportunity to comprehend segment size. If you purchase a container of pop from the store, you'll presumably drink every last bit of it. The jug is a piece.

Yet, the container probably won't be a solitary serve. While contrasting the supplement content of food varieties, it's consistently critical to take a gander at the serving size to guarantee that you're contrasting one type with its logical counterpart.

Past its convenience for making examinations, understanding the idea of part size can likewise be the most important phase in rolling out serious improvements to your eating regimen. Segment sizes have gotten bigger over the long haul. Individuals eat more servings at a time. By diminishing part size, you can in any case have a portion of your old top choices while bringing down the glucose you're consuming.

Counting carbs:
With this strategy, understanding serving size versus segment size is particularly significant. For every feast, you want to take a gander at the nourishing data for the food you're eating and monitor the complete number of starches you eat with every dinner.

How much carbs you can have per dinner changes depending upon a few variables, including age, weight, and activity level. As a common rule, the CDC[1] suggests that individuals with diabetes get about a portion of their everyday calories from carbs.

While counting carbs, it's essential to comprehend which ones can build your glucose. Your nutritional mark will most likely break the starches segment into three classifications: fiber, sugar, and added sugar.

As we've seen, starch is likewise a carb, however, that frequently is excluded from dietary names. Sugar (added or regular) and starch both raise your glucose, but fiber doesn't. Thus, just deducting the grams of fiber from the grams of all-out carbs will give you the starch count that can increment glucose.

The plating strategy:
However long you're cautious with serving sizes and precisely record every one of the starches you consume, counting carbs is a superb technique to work out carbs consumed. In any case, it isn't the most helpful. This is particularly valid for those who are simply starting to make changes to their way of life to assist with overseeing diabetes.

The plating strategy is a more straightforward approach to overseeing carbs that might function admirably enough for you, basically to begin on the way to creating better dietary patterns. For the plate strategy, you start with a 9-inch supper plate.

Chapter 3

How might I forestall diabetes?

Type 1 diabetes can't be forestalled. However, the sound way of life decisions that help treat prediabetes, type 2 diabetes, and gestational diabetes can likewise assist with forestalling them:

Eat quality food varieties. Pick food varieties lower in fat and calories and higher in fiber. Center around natural products, vegetables, and entire grains. Eat an assortment to hold back from feeling exhausted.

Get more active work. Attempt to get around 30 minutes of moderate high-impact movement on most days of the week. Or on the other hand, plan to get something like 150 minutes of moderate oxygen-consuming action in seven days. For instance, go for a lively everyday stroll. If you can't fit in a long exercise, split it up into more modest meetings over the day.

Lose abundance of pounds. On the off chance that you're overweight, losing even 7% of your body weight can bring down the gamble of diabetes. For instance, assuming that you weigh 200 pounds (90.7 kilograms), shedding 14 pounds (6.4 kilograms) can bring down the gamble of diabetes.

However, don't attempt to get fitter during pregnancy. Converse with your supplier about how much weight is good for you to acquire during pregnancy.

To keep your weight within a sound reach, work on long-haul changes to your eating and exercise propensities. Recall the advantages of getting in shape, like a better heart, more energy, and higher confidence.

Now and again sedates are a choice. Oral diabetes medications like metformin (Glumetza, Fortamet, others) may bring down the gamble of type 2 diabetes. Yet, solid way-of-life decisions are significant. If you have prediabetes, have your glucose looked at no less than once every year to ensure you haven't created type 2 diabetes?

Chapter 4

Some breakfast meal recipes for diabetics;
Two-Ingredient Banana Pancakes:

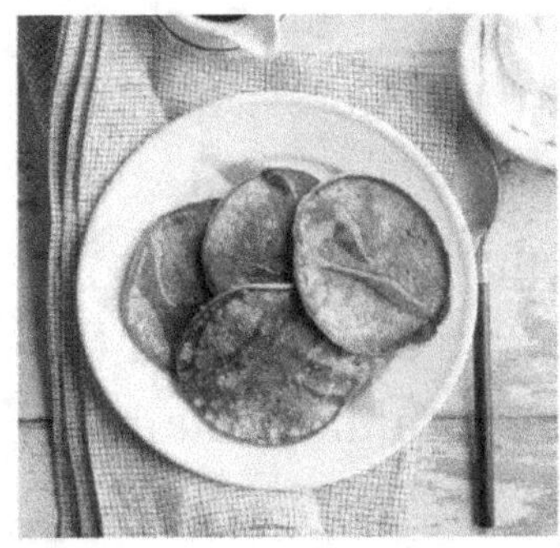

These delicious and unbelievably simple
pancakes are best enjoyed right after cooking.
With just eggs and a banana, you can have
healthy grain-free pancakes with no added sugar.
Serve with maple syrup and yogurt or ricotta
cheese to add in some protein.

Ingredients
2 large eggs
1 medium banana
Directions

Step 1

Puree eggs and banana in a blender until smooth.

Step 2

Lightly oil a large nonstick skillet and heat over medium heat. Using 2 tablespoons of batter for each pancake, drop 4 mounds of batter into the pan. Cook until bubbles appear on the surface and the edges look dry, 2 to 4 minutes. Using a thin spatula, gently flip the pancakes and cook until browned on the bottom, 1 to 2 minutes more. Transfer the pancakes to a plate. Lightly oil the pan again and repeat with the remaining batter.

Nutrition Facts

Serving Size: 4 pancakes

Per Serving: 124 calories; protein 6.9g; carbohydrates 13.8g; dietary fiber 1.5g; sugars 7.4g; fat 4.9g; saturated fat 1.6g; cholesterol 186 mg; vitamin a iu 307.8IU; vitamin c 5.1mg; folate 35.3mcg; calcium 31mg; iron 1mg; magnesium 21.9mg; potassium 280.2mg; sodium 71.6mg.

Exchanges: 1 fruit, 1 medium-fat

Spinach & Egg Scramble with Raspberries:

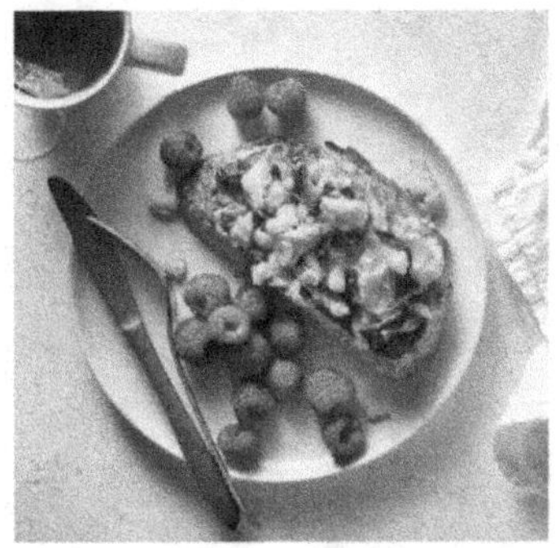

This quick egg scramble with hearty bread is one of the best breakfasts for weight loss. It combines protein-packed eggs and superfood raspberries with filling whole-grain toast and nutrient-rich spinach. The protein and fiber help fill you up and keep you going through the morning.

Ingredients

1 teaspoon canola oil

1 ½ cups baby spinach (1 1/2 ounces)

2 large eggs, lightly beaten

Pinch of kosher salt

Pinch of ground pepper

1 slice whole-grain bread, toasted

½ cup fresh raspberries

Directions
Step 1
Heat oil in a small nonstick skillet over medium-high heat. Add spinach and cook until wilted, stirring often, 1 to 2 minutes. Transfer the spinach to a plate. Wipe the pan clean, place over medium heat and add eggs.Cook, stirring once or twice to ensure even cooking, until just set, 1 to 2 minutes. Stir in the spinach, salt and pepper. Serve the scramble with toast and raspberries.
Nutrition Facts:

Serving Size: 2 eggs, 1 slice bread & 1/2 cup raspberries

Per Serving: 296 calories; protein 17.8g; carbohydrates 20.9g; dietary fiber 7g; sugars 4.8g; fat 15.7g; saturated fat 3.7g; cholesterol 372mg; vitamin a iu 3312.6IU; vitamin c 28.1mg; folate 79.4mcg; calcium 138.8mg; iron 4.2mg; magnesium 76.1mg; potassium 292.6mg; sodium 394.2mg; thiamin 0.1mg.
Exchanges: 2 medium-fat protein, 1 fat, 1/2 fruit, 1/2 starch, 1/2 vegetable

Pistachio & Peach Toast;

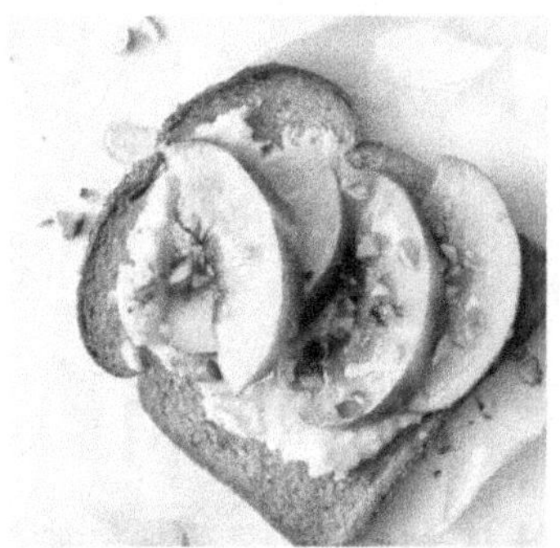

This breakfast is great when you have leftover ricotta cheese--plus it comes together in just 5 minutes

Ingredients

1 tablespoon part-skim ricotta cheese

1 teaspoon honey, divided

⅛ teaspoon cinnamon

1 slice 100% whole-wheat bread, toasted

½ medium peach, sliced

1 tablespoon chopped pistachios

Directions
Step 1
Combine ricotta, ½ teaspoon honey and cinnamon in a small bowl.

Step 2
Spread the ricotta mixture on toast and top with peach and pistachios. Drizzle with the remaining 1/2 teaspoon honey.

Nutrition Facts

Serving Size: 1 toast

Per Serving: 193 calories; protein 8.2g; carbohydrates 29g; dietary fiber 3.9g; sugars 13.9g; fat 6g; saturated fat 1.4g; cholesterol 4.8mg; vitamin a iu 326.4IU; vitamin c 5.2mg; folate 22.1mcg; calcium 91.1mg; iron 1.4mg; magnesium 42.5mg; potassium 325.8mg; sodium 157.4mg; added sugar 5.8g.

Peanut Butter-Banana English Muffin:

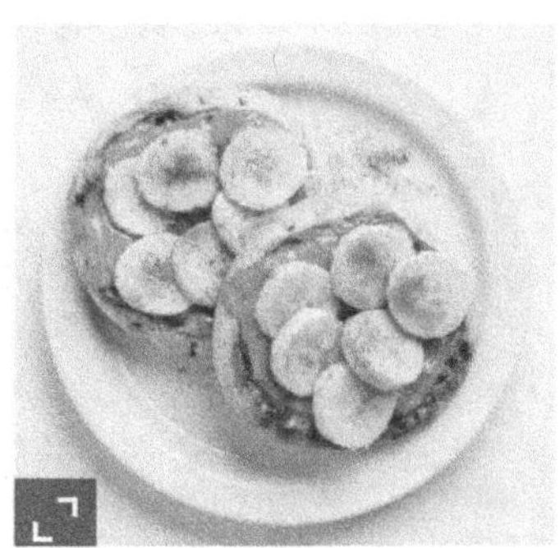

Peanut butter and banana are the original power couple. Top a simple toasted English muffin with the duo, then sprinkle everything with a hit of ground cinnamon for a healthy breakfast of champions

Ingredients

1 whole-wheat English muffin, toasted

1 tablespoon peanut butter

½ banana, sliced

Pinch of ground cinnamon

Directions
Step 1
Top English muffin with peanut butter, banana and cinnamon.
Nutrition Facts
Serving Size: 1 serving
Per Serving: 344 calories; protein 10.6g; carbohydrates 56.8g; dietary fiber 8.6g; sugars 20.3g; fat 9.8g; saturated fat 1.6g; vitamin a iu 79.3IU; vitamin c 10.3mg; folate 56 mcg; calcium 182.4mg; iron 2.1mg; magnesium

78.8mg; potassium 561.7mg; sodium 293.9mg; added sugar 5g.
Exchanges: 1 1/2 starch, 1 1/2 high-fat protein, 1 fruit

Breakfast Salad with Egg & Salsa Verde Vinaigrette:

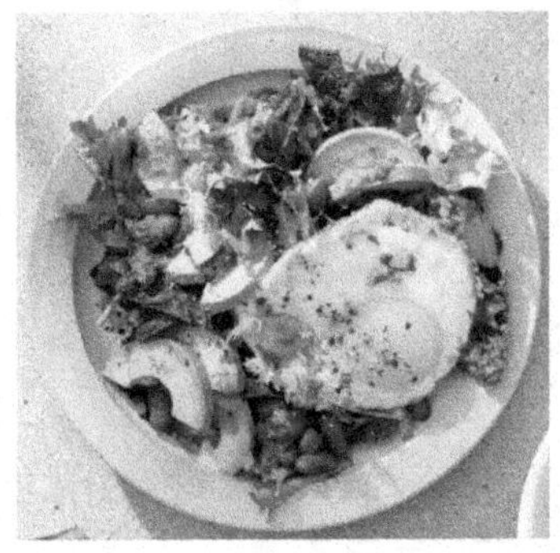

Salad for breakfast? Don't knock it until you've tried it. We love how this meal gives you 3 whole cups of vegetables to start your day.

Ingredients

3 tablespoons salsa verde, such as Frontera brand

1 tablespoon plus 1 tsp. extra-virgin olive oil, divided

2 tablespoons chopped cilantro, plus more for garnish

2 cups mesclun or other salad greens

8 blue corn tortilla chips, broken into large pieces

½ cup canned red kidney beans, rinsed

¼ avocado, sliced

1 large egg

Directions:

Step 1
Whisk salsa, 1 Tbsp. oil, and cilantro in a small bowl. Toss half the mixture with mesclun (or other greens) in a shallow dinner bowl.

Step 2
Layer chips, beans, and avocado atop the salad.

Step 3
Heat the remaining 1 tsp. oil in a small nonstick
skillet over medium-high heat. Add egg and fry
until the white is completely cooked but the yolk
is still slightly runny, about 2 minutes.

Step 4
Serve the egg on the salad. Drizzle with the
remaining salsa vinaigrette and sprinkle with
additional cilantro, if desired.

Nutrition Facts:
Serving Size: 3 cups salad + 1 egg + 5 Tbsp.
vinaigrette
Per Serving: 527 calories; protein 16g;
carbohydrates 37g; dietary fiber 13g; sugars 2g;
fat 34g; saturated fat 5g; cholesterol 186 mg;
potassium 1001mg; sodium 660mg.

Scrambled Eggs with Sausage:

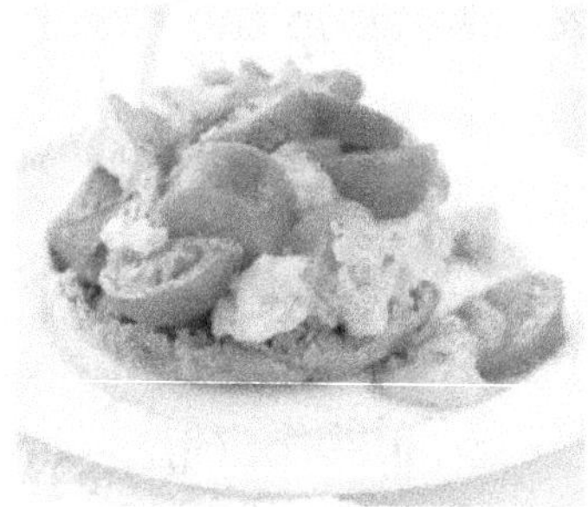

Start your day off right with these scrambled eggs. This recipe includes eggs, turkey sausage, and cheese; packing 14 grams of protein per serving. Quick and easy to make, this is the perfect breakfast solution.

Ingredients

Nonstick cooking spray

2 eggs

2 tablespoons reduced-sodium chicken broth

Ground black pepper

1 ounce cooked turkey sausage, sliced

¼ cup cherry tomatoes, quartered

2 tablespoons finely shredded reduced-fat Cheddar cheese

1 whole-grain English muffin, halved and toasted
Directions:

Step 1
Coat a large nonstick skillet with cooking spray. Preheat the skillet over medium heat.

Step 2
In a medium bowl, use a whisk or rotary beater to beat together eggs, broth and black pepper; stir in sliced sausage.

Step 3
Pour egg mixture into a hot skillet. Cook over medium heat, without stirring, until mixture begins to set on the bottom and around edges.

Step 4

With a spatula or a large spoon, lift and fold the partially cooked egg mixture so the uncooked portion flows underneath. Continue cooking over medium heat until almost set; add tomatoes and cheese. Cook about 1 minute more or until egg mixture is cooked through but is still glossy and moist.

Step 5

Serve over toasted English muffin halves.

Nutrition Facts;

Serving Size: 1 english muffin half and 1 1/2 cups egg mixture
Per Serving: 198 calories; protein 14.5g; carbohydrates 15.6g; dietary fiber 2.5g; sugars 4.3g; fat 9.3g; saturated fat 3.1g; cholesterol 230.5mg; vitamin a iu 507.8IU; vitamin c 2.9mg; folate 44.3mcg; calcium 222mg; iron 2.1mg; magnesium 38.5mg; potassium 244.4mg; sodium 523.7mg

Chapter 5

Slow-Cooker Braised Beef with Carrots & Turnips;

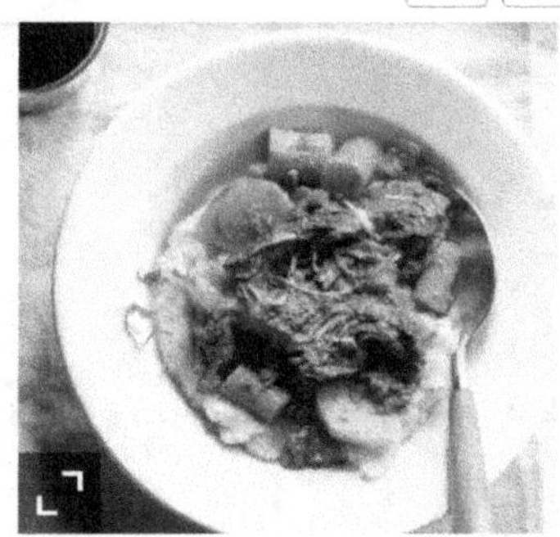

The spice blend in this healthy beef stew recipe—cinnamon, allspice and cloves—may conjure images of apple pie, but the combo is a great fit in savory applications too. Serve over creamy polenta or buttered whole-wheat egg noodles.

Ingredients

1 tablespoon kosher salt

2 teaspoons ground cinnamon

½ teaspoon ground allspice

½ teaspoon ground pepper

¼ teaspoon ground cloves

3-3 1/2 pounds beef chuck roast, trimmed

2 tablespoons extra-virgin olive oil

1 medium onion, chopped

3 cloves garlic, sliced

1 cup red wine

1 (28 ounce) can whole tomatoes, preferably San Marzano

5 medium carrots, cut into 1-inch pieces

2 medium turnips, peeled and cut into 1/2-inch pieces

Chopped fresh basil for garnish

Directions

Step 1
Combine salt, cinnamon, allspice, pepper and cloves in a small bowl. Rub the mixture all over the beef.

Step 2
Heat oil in a large skillet over medium heat. Add the beef and cook until browned, 4 to 5 minutes per side. Transfer to a 5- to 6-quart slow cooker.

Step 3
Add onion and garlic to the pan. Cook, stirring, for 2 minutes. Add wine and tomatoes (with their juice); bring to a boil, scraping up any browned bits and breaking up the tomatoes. Add the mixture to the slow cooker along with carrots and turnips.

Step 4

Cover and cook on High for 4 hours or Low for
8 hours.

Step 5

Remove the beef from the slow cooker and slice.
Serve the beef with the sauce and vegetables,
garnished with basil, if desired.

Tips

Active: 40 minutes Slow-cooker time: 4-8 hours

To make ahead: Refrigerate the browned beef
(Steps 1-2) and tomato mixture (Step 3)
separately for up to 1 day. Bring the tomato
mixture to a boil before adding to the slow
cooker.

Equipment: 5- to 6-quart slow cooker

Nutrition Facts;

Serving Size: 3 oz. beef & 1 cup vegetables each

Per Serving: 318 calories; protein 34.7g; carbohydrates 12.8g; dietary fiber 3.1g; sugars 6.2g; fat 10.7g; saturated fat 3.2g; cholesterol 98.9mg; vitamin a iu 6776.9IU; vitamin c 17.4mg; folate 26.3mcg; calcium 69mg; iron 3.5mg; magnesium 36mg; potassium 697.7mg; sodium 538.4mg.

Exchanges: 2 vegetable, 4 1/2 lean meat, 1/2 fat

Cream of Turkey & Wild Rice Soup;

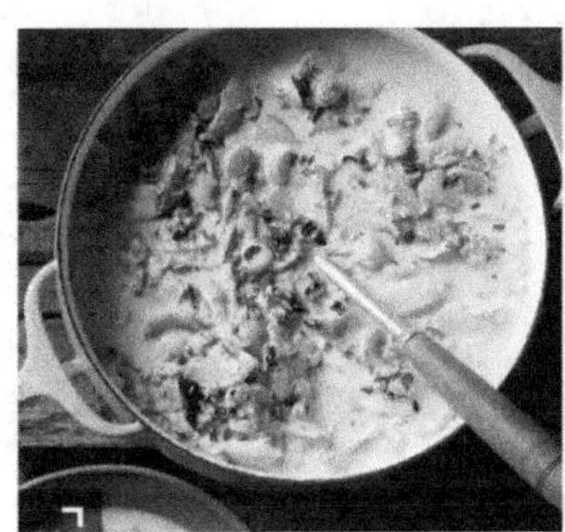

Got leftover cooked chicken or turkey? Cook up a pot of soup! This low-sodium soup recipe is a healthier twist on a classic creamy turkey and wild rice soup that hails from Minnesota. Serve

with a crisp romaine salad and whole-grain
bread.

Ingredients

1 tablespoon extra-virgin olive oil

2 cups sliced mushrooms, (about 4 ounces)

¾ cup chopped celery

¾ cup chopped carrots

¼ cup chopped shallots

¼ cup all-purpose flour

¼ teaspoon salt

¼ teaspoon freshly ground pepper

4 cups reduced-sodium chicken broth

1 cup quick-cooking or instant wild rice, (see Ingredient Note)

3 cups shredded cooked chicken, or turkey (12 ounces; see Tip)

½ cup reduced-fat sour cream

2 tablespoons chopped fresh parsley

Directions;
Step 1
Heat oil in a large saucepan over medium heat. Add mushrooms, celery, carrots and shallots; cook, stirring, until softened, about 5 minutes. Add flour, salt and pepper; cook, stirring, for 2 minutes more.

Step 2
Add broth and bring to a boil, scraping up any browned bits. Add rice and reduce heat to a simmer. Cover and cook until the rice is tender, 5 to 7 minutes. Stir in turkey (or chicken), sour

cream and parsley; cook until heated through, about 2 minutes more

Ingredient note;
Quick-cooking or instant wild rice has been parboiled to reduce the cooking time. Conventional wild rice takes 40 to 50 minutes to cook. Be sure to check the cooking directions when selecting your rice--some brands labeled "quick" take about 30 minutes to cook. If you can't find the quick-cooking variety, just add cooked conventional wild rice along with the turkey at the end of Step 2.

Tip:
To poach chicken breasts, place boneless, skinless chicken breasts in a medium skillet or saucepan. Add lightly salted water to cover and bring to a boil. Cover, reduce heat to low and simmer gently until chicken is cooked through and no longer pink in the middle, 10 to 12 minutes.

Nutrition Facts;

Serving Size: about 1 3/4 cups

Per Serving: 378 calories; protein 36.9g; carbohydrates 28.5g; dietary fiber 2.7g; sugars 2.8g; fat 10.6g; saturated fat 3.7g; cholesterol 79.7mg; vitamin a iu 4518.3IU; vitamin c 6.3mg; folate 57.3mcg; calcium 73.2mg; iron 2.4mg; magnesium 45.7mg; potassium 748.3mg; sodium 364.1mg; thiamin 0.2mg.

Exchanges: 1 1/2 starch, 1 vegetable, 3 lean meat,

Sheet-Pan Chicken Fajita Bowls;

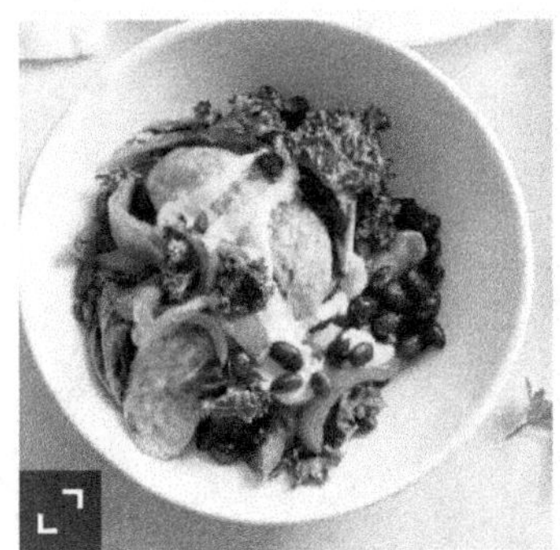

Skip the tortillas in favor of this warm fajita salad, which features a nutritious medley of chicken with roasted kale, bell peppers and black beans. The chicken, beans and vegetables are all cooked in the same pan, so this healthy dinner is easy to make and the cleanup is easy too.

Ingredients;

2 teaspoons chili powder

2 teaspoons ground cumin

¾ teaspoon salt, divided

½ teaspoon garlic powder

½ teaspoon smoked paprika

¼ teaspoon ground pepper

2 tablespoons olive oil, divided

1 ¼ pounds chicken tenders

1 medium yellow onion, sliced

1 medium red bell pepper, sliced

1 medium green bell pepper, sliced

4 cups chopped stemmed kale

1 (15 ounce) can no-salt-added black beans, rinsed

¼ cup low-fat plain Greek yogurt

1 tablespoon lime juice

2 teaspoons water

Directions:
Step 1
Place a large rimmed baking sheet in the oven; preheat to 425 degrees F.
Step 2
Combine chili powder, cumin, 1/2 tsp. salt, garlic powder, paprika, and ground pepper in a large bowl. Transfer 1 tsp. of the spice mixture to a medium bowl and set aside. Whisk 1 Tbsp.

oil into the remaining spice mixture in the large bowl. Add chicken, onion, and red and green bell peppers; toss to coat.

Step 3
Remove the pan from the oven; coat with cooking spray. Spread the chicken mixture in an even layer on the pan. Roast for 15 minutes.

Step 4
Meanwhile, combine kale and black beans with the remaining 1/4 tsp. salt and 1 Tbsp. olive oil in a large bowl; toss to coat.

Step 5
Remove the pan from the oven. Stir the chicken and vegetables. Spread kale and beans evenly over the top. Roast until the chicken is cooked through and the vegetables are tender, 5 to 7 minutes more.

Step 6
Meanwhile, add yogurt, lime juice, and water to the reserved spice mixture; stir to combine.

Step 7
Divide the chicken and vegetable mixture among
4 bowls. Drizzle with the yogurt dressing and
serve.

Tips
Tip: For easier weeknight prep, slice vegetables
the night before; cover and refrigerate.

To make ahead: Prepare spice mixture (Step 1)
up to 2 days ahead; store in an airtight container.

Nutrition Facts
Serving Size: 2 chicken tenders, 1 1/4 cups
vegetables + generous 1 Tbsp. sauce
Per Serving: 343 calories; protein 42.7g;
carbohydrates 23.7g; dietary fiber 8.2g; sugars
3.8g; fat 9.9g; saturated fat 1.4g; cholesterol
70.9mg; vitamin a iu 2774.9IU; vitamin c
72.9mg; folate 25.3mcg; calcium 187.3mg; iron
3.6mg; magnesium 62.7mg; potassium 579.8mg;
sodium 605.1mg.

Vegan White Bean Chili;

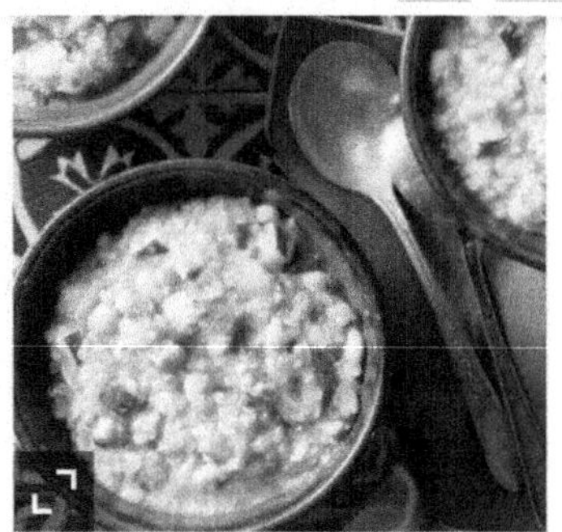

Fresh Anaheim (or poblano) chiles add mild heat to this classic white bean chili and contribute lots of smoky flavor. Quinoa adds body to the chili, while diced zucchini provides pretty flecks of green and increases the veggie content.

Ingredients;

¼ cup avocado oil or canola oil

2 cups chopped seeded Anaheim or poblano chiles (about 3)

1 large onion, chopped

4 cloves garlic, minced

½ cup quinoa, rinsed

4 teaspoons dried oregano

4 teaspoons ground cumin

1 teaspoon salt

½ teaspoon ground coriander

½ teaspoon ground pepper

4 cups low-sodium vegetable broth

2 (15 ounce) cans no-salt-added white beans, rinsed

1 large zucchini, diced (about 3 cups)

¼ cup chopped fresh cilantro

2 tablespoons lime juice, plus wedges for
serving

Directions;
Step 1
Heat oil in a large pot over medium heat. Add
chiles, onion and garlic. Cook, stirring, until the
vegetables are softened, 5 to 7 minutes. Add
quinoa, oregano, cumin, salt, coriander and
pepper; cook, stirring, until aromatic, about 1
minute. Stir in broth and beans. Bring to a boil.
Reduce heat to a simmer. Partially cover and
cook, stirring occasionally, for 20 minutes. Add
zucchini; cover and continue cooking until the
zucchini is soft and the chili has thickened, 10 to
15 minutes more. Stir in cilantro and lime juice.
Serve with lime wedges, if desired.

Tips
To make ahead: Refrigerate chili for up to 4
days. Reheat before serving

Nutrition Facts;
Serving Size: 1 1/3 cups

Per Serving: 283 calories; protein 9.7g; carbohydrates 36.7g; dietary fiber 8.4g; sugars 6.6g; fat 11.7g; saturated fat 1.3g; vitamin a iu 757.3IU; vitamin c 135.4mg; folate 77.7mcg; calcium 96.4mg; iron 3.9mg; magnesium 107.6mg; potassium 670.7mg; sodium 529.4mg; thiamin 0.7mg.
Exchanges: 2 fat, 2 vegetable, 1 1/2 starch, 1/2 lean protein

Paprika Baked Pork Tenderloin with Potatoes & Broccoli;

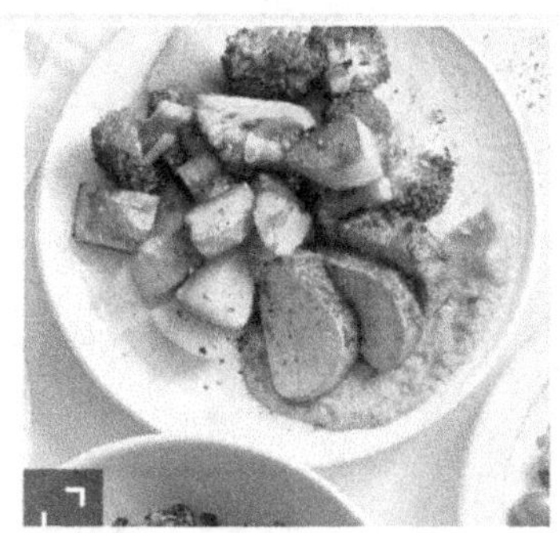

You'd never guess that this elegant meal comes together on just one baking sheet. While the pork rests, whip together an easy red pepper sauce to complete this impressive and healthy dinner. The sauce would also be delicious with chicken.

We're willing to bet this easy sheet-pan dinner recipe will go into heavy rotation on your kitchen playlist.

Ingredients

¾ pound Yukon Gold potatoes, scrubbed and cut into 1-inch pieces

1 medium red onion, cut into 1 inch pieces

2 tablespoons olive oil, divided

¾ teaspoon salt, divided

4 cups broccoli florets (about 1 lb.)

2 cloves garlic, peeled

1 ½ teaspoons smoked paprika

½ teaspoon ground pepper, divided

2 teaspoons Dijon mustard

1 (1 pound) pork tenderloin, trimmed

2 jarred roasted red bell peppers (6 oz.)

2 tablespoons low-fat sour cream or low-fat
plain Greek yogurt

1 teaspoon lemon juice
Directions;
Step 1
Place a large rimmed baking sheet in the oven;
preheat to 425 degrees F.

Step 2
Combine potatoes, onion, 1 Tbsp. oil, and 1/4
tsp. salt in a medium bowl; toss to coat. Remove
the pan from the oven; coat with cooking spray.
Spread the potato mixture on the pan; roast for
15 minutes.

Step 3
Meanwhile, combine broccoli, 2 tsp. olive oil,
and 1/4 tsp. salt in a medium bowl; toss to coat.

Place garlic on a small piece of foil. Drizzle with
the remaining 1 tsp. oil; fold up into a small
packet. Combine paprika, 1/4 tsp. ground
pepper, and the remaining 1/4 tsp. salt in a small
bowl. Spread mustard all over pork. Coat with
the paprika mixture.

Step 4

Remove the pan from the oven. Stir the potatoes
and onions and move them to one side. Place the
pork next to the potatoes; spread the broccoli on
the other side of the pan. Place the packet of
garlic where there is space. Roast until an
instant-read thermometer inserted in the thickest
part of the pork registers reaches 145 degrees F,
about 25 minutes.

Step 5

Let the pork rest while you make the sauce:
Carefully unwrap the garlic and transfer it to a
mini food processor or blender. Add roasted red
peppers, sour cream (or yogurt), lemon juice,
and the remaining 1/4 tsp. ground pepper. Puree
until smooth.

Step 6
Cut the pork into 12 slices. Divide the pork,
potatoes, and broccoli among 4 plates. Drizzle
the red pepper sauce over the top.

Nutrition Facts;
Per Serving: 323 calories; protein 30g;
carbohydrates 28.7g; dietary fiber 5.3g; sugars
5.5g; fat 10.3g; saturated fat 2.1g; cholesterol
76.2mg; vitamin a iu 3879.9IU; vitamin c 154
mg; folate 98.4mcg; calcium 98.9mg; iron
3.2mg; magnesium 83.8mg; potassium
1246.8mg; sodium 730.7mg.

Lemon-Garlic Pasta with Salmon;

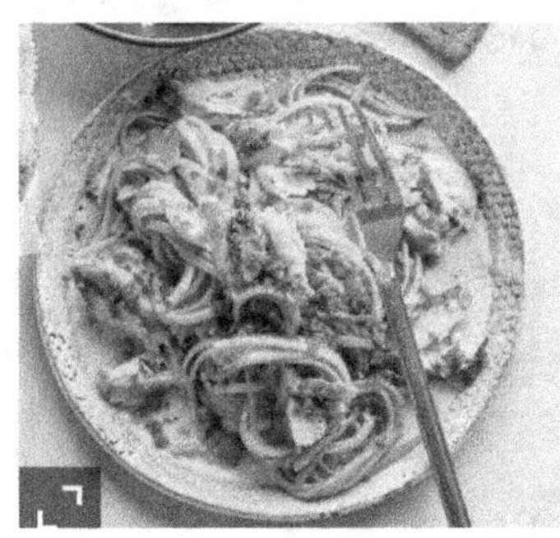

Wondering what to do with leftover salmon? This is a delicious and easy way to turn it into another weeknight-friendly, quick dinner. Don't forget to reserve some pasta water—its starch thickens the lemon-garlic pasta sauce and makes it silky-smooth.

Ingredients;

8 ounces whole-wheat pasta

5 tablespoons extra-virgin olive oil

5 cloves garlic, chopped

1 teaspoon anchovy paste

¼ teaspoon crushed red pepper

Zest and juice of 1 lemon

1 1/2 cups flaked cooked salmon

3 tablespoons chopped fresh parsley

¼ teaspoon salt

2 tablespoons whole-wheat breadcrumbs, toasted

Directions;
Step 1
Cook pasta according to package directions.
Drain, reserving 1/2 cup cooking water.

Step 2
Combine oil, garlic, anchovy paste, crushed red
pepper, lemon zest and lemon juice in a large
skillet. Heat over medium-high heat until
sizzling, about 3 minutes. Add the reserved
water, the pasta, salmon, parsley and salt. Cook,
stirring, until the sauce coats the pasta, about 2
minutes. Serve topped with breadcrumbs.

Nutrition Facts;
Serving Size: 1 1/3 cup
Per Serving: 473 calories; protein 19.8g;
carbohydrates 49.4g; dietary fiber 5.9g; sugars
3.6g; fat 23g; saturated fat 3.4g; cholesterol

25.5mg; vitamin a iu 366.8IU; vitamin c 16.2mg; folate 59.2mcg; calcium 63.1mg; iron 2.8mg; magnesium 93.9mg; potassium 513 mg; sodium 394.9mg; added sugar 1g.
Exchanges: 3 1/2 fat, 3 starch, 1 1/2 lean protein

THE END